UNDERSTANDING BIOFEEDBACK THERAPY

Harnessing Your Body's Signals For Holistic Healing, Wellness, Enhancing Your Mind-Body Connection And More

DR. KARSON BRYAN

Copyright © 2023, Dr. Karson Bryan

DISCLAIMER

This book's content is meant to be used solely for general informative purposes. Despite having taken every precaution to guarantee the content's accuracy, the author disclaims all duty and responsibility for any errors or omissions. It is recommended that readers exercise caution and, if needed, seek expert guidance. Any and all liability for losses, damages, or other outcomes arising from the use of the material included in this book is disclaimed by the author and publisher. All referenced product names and trademarks are the property of their respective owners and are merely cited for identification. Any likeness to real people or things is entirely accidental. Since it is a work of fiction, this book should not be used as a substitute for professional, legal, or medical advice. It is advised that readers seek advice on particular issues from qualified experts."

Please make sure that this disclaimer is modified to fit the particular requirements and subject matter of your book. Seeking advice from a legal expert is also a smart option if you have any questions or require a more thorough disclaimer for your specific book.

TABLE OF CONTENTS

CHAPTER ONE

BIOFEEDBACK THERAPY

INTRODUCTION

An intriguing area of medicine that has grown in popularity and attention recently is biofeedback therapy. It entails utilizing technology to give people more control over their body's physiological processes, including heart rate, muscle tension, and brainwave activity. By giving people access to real-time information on their physiological processes, this therapy method has the potential to enhance general health and well-being by empowering people to make conscious changes and improve their self-regulation.

DESCRIBE BIOFEEDBACK

Biofeedback is a treatment approach that gives people real-time information on their physiological processes using electronic monitoring devices. Information about generally involuntary body functions, such as heart rate, skin temperature, muscular tension, and brainwave activity, is included in this data. Increasing a person's awareness of these physiological processes and giving them the ability to voluntarily regulate them is the main objective of biofeedback. People who are trying to improve their general well-being or who are coping with a variety of medical issues may find that this increased control is really helpful.

BIOFEEDBACK THERAPY'S PAST

The origins of biofeedback therapy can be found in the late 1960s when physicians and researchers started investigating the possibility of giving people feedback about their physiological processes through electrical devices. Neal Miller and Elmer Green were early pioneers in this subject, having pioneered important research on biofeedback techniques. The field of biofeedback therapy developed further in the ensuing decades as a result of the creation of increasingly sophisticated monitoring tools and an expanding corpus of studies demonstrating its efficacy.

Biofeedback treatment has been used over the years to treat a wide range of physiological and psychological issues, such as anxiety, chronic pain, stress reduction, and other health issues. This therapy's adaptability has made it a useful resource for medical professionals as well as those looking for non-invasive, drug-free approaches to improve their health and well-being.

BIOFEEDBACK'S OPERATION

Physiological data is measured and recorded using a variety of sensors and devices in biofeedback systems. These sensors are affixed to the subject's body, and a monitoring device receives the data they gather. Feedback is usually given in the form of visual or aural signals that convey current information about the particular physiological activity being watched, like a graph on a computer screen, a tone, or a light.

People are urged to use this knowledge to become more in tune with their bodies and learn how to consciously modify them to reach a desired condition. When using biofeedback for stress management, for instance, a person might observe on a monitor how their heart rate rises in reaction to stress and then learn how to lower it using strategies like deep breathing or relaxation exercises.

People can learn to self-regulate their physiological processes and better manage their situations over time with practice and encouragement.

Biofeedback treatment is an effective strategy for enhancing health and well-being that makes use of the power of physiological feedback that occurs in real-time.

CHAPTER TWO

BIOFEEDBACK TYPES

The biofeedback technique known as electromyography (EMG) is centered on the monitoring and reporting of muscle activity. This method measures the electrical activity produced by muscle contractions by implanting electrodes or sensors into the skin or straight into the muscles. Muscle tension and relaxation can be evaluated and trained using electromyography (EMG). People can learn to understand and regulate their muscle activity by monitoring the electrical signals generated by their muscle contractions.

MUSCLE TENSION AND RELAXATION

People can learn muscle relaxation techniques and become more conscious of their muscle tension with the help of EMG biofeedback. EMG gives people immediate feedback on their muscular activity, which helps them understand how stress, worry, or tension impairs their ability to use their muscles. With this knowledge, they can create relaxation techniques to ease tense muscles, including progressive muscle relaxation, deep breathing exercises, or mindfulness. People can improve their capacity to consciously regulate muscular activity by regular practice and feedback, which will ultimately result in a decrease in tension and discomfort.

APPLICATIONS AND BENEFITS

There are several real-world uses for EMG biofeedback. It is frequently used in therapeutic settings to treat a variety of muscle pain issues, including back and neck pain, temporomandibular joint (TMJ) disorders, and tension headaches. Additionally, it can be used in rehabilitation programs to help patients heal after surgeries or injuries that impair muscle function. Moreover, EMG biofeedback has been used in sports training to enhance athletes' performance and muscular control.

Furthermore, EMG biofeedback helps people better control their body's physiological reactions to stress, which makes it useful in treating diseases associated with stress. Through the practice of muscular relaxation, individuals can lessen the detrimental effects of ongoing stress on their general health. EMG biofeedback is a flexible tool in the field of biofeedback since it is a safe, non-invasive technique that can be used to supplement other therapeutic approaches.

ELECTROENCEPHALOGRAPHY

Another well-known biofeedback method that tracks brainwave activity is electroencephalography (EEG). Electrodes are applied to the scalp to measure the electrical signals produced by brain neurons in the EEG. These signals are divided into several brainwave kinds, including beta, gamma, theta, alpha, and beta waves, each of which is connected to a certain mental state and cognitive function.

BRAINWAVE ACTIVITY

EEG biofeedback, sometimes referred to as neurofeedback, provides people with up-to-date knowledge on their brainwave activity. People can learn more about their mental health, level of focus, and level of relaxation by examining the patterns in their brainwave frequencies.

For instance, higher alpha wave activity is connected to a calm and contemplative state, whereas higher beta wave activity is connected to alertness and cognitive activity. Neurofeedback trains people to optimize and control their brainwave patterns, which help them reach targeted mental states and cognitive improvements.

COGNITIVE ENHANCEMENTS AND NEUROFEEDBACK

As a subsection of EEG biofeedback, neurofeedback has drawn interest due to its potential to improve mental health and cognitive performance. People can learn to alter their brainwave patterns to increase focus, lower anxiety, and elevate their mood through neurofeedback training.

Applications for this strategy include managing attention-deficit/hyperactivity disorder (ADHD), reducing anxiety and stress, and even helping athletes, artists, and professionals reach their top performance.

The cognitive improvements attained by neurofeedback training are frequently customized, with training regimens made to meet the unique requirements and objectives of each participant.

CHAPTER THREE

VARIABILITY IN HEALTH RATES

HEART-RELATED HEALTH

Heart Rate Variability, which is a measurement of the difference in time between successive heartbeats, is closely related to cardiovascular health. It is a useful marker of the health of the autonomic nervous system and can be an effective instrument for evaluating cardiovascular function. Superior cardiovascular health is typically linked to a larger heart rate variability. It represents an autonomic nerve system that is adaptable to different demands and pressures. Conversely, low HRV may be a sign of an overreaction to stress, which has been connected to a higher risk of heart disease.

STRESS REDUCTION

One important use of HRV is stress management. The sympathetic and parasympathetic nervous systems' equilibrium is reflected in HRV, which offers information on how a person's body reacts to stress. Reduced heart rate variability (HRV) is a sign of high-stress levels and the predominance of the sympathetic (fight-or-flight) response. HRV can be raised by practicing mindfulness, relaxation, and other stress management skills. This can enhance cardiovascular health and general well-being.

SKIN TEMPERATURE AND CONDUCTANCE

Important markers of stress and emotional reactions include skin conductance and temperature. The electrical conductivity of the skin is measured by skin conductance, which is a reflection of sympathetic nervous system activity. It is frequently used to measure stress levels and emotional reactions in conjunction with HRV. Elevated skin conductance could be a result of an elevated stress reaction.

On the other hand, changes in peripheral blood flow that are mediated by the autonomic nervous system can be indicated by variations in skin temperature. Peripheral vasoconstriction, a result of the body's "fight or flight" reaction during stress or worry, can lower skin temperature. Through the use of temperature and skin conductance data, biofeedback can assist people in becoming more conscious of their stress reactions and developing efficient coping mechanisms.

REDUCING STRESS AND ANXIETY

Techniques for reducing stress and anxiety can have a big impact on HRV and general health. Deep breathing, yoga, meditation, and biofeedback are a few practices that people can use to regulate their autonomic nervous system and raise their heart rate variability (HRV). By encouraging a more balanced sympathetic and parasympathetic response, these techniques help lower the likelihood of long-term stress and the health issues that go along with it.

BIOFEEDBACK IN DISORDERS OF THE SKIN

The field of "biofeedback in skin disorders" is a young one that uses HRV monitoring and other biofeedback techniques to treat skin diseases like dermatitis, psoriasis, and eczema. These issues are greatly exacerbated by stress, and biofeedback can help people better control their stress reactions, which will ultimately enhance the health of their skin. People can learn more about the physiological and mental states that influence their skin disorders and develop more effective treatment and management strategies by tracking their heart rate variability (HRV) and other physiological indicators.

Heart rate variability is a useful metric for evaluating stress reduction, cardiovascular health, and general well-being.

CHAPTER FOUR

CONDITIONS BIOFEEDBACK IS USED TO TREAT

A treatment strategy called biofeedback aids people in becoming conscious of and in charge of their bodily physiological processes. Patients can learn how to control these processes for improved health and well-being by using monitoring devices to offer real-time information about a variety of body systems. Although there are many medical disorders for which biofeedback can be used, this book will go into great detail on how it can be used to manage chronic pain, with a special emphasis on musculoskeletal pain, migraines, and headaches.

MANAGEMENT OF CHRONIC PAIN

A person's quality of life can be greatly impacted by chronic pain, which is a persistent and frequently incapacitating ailment. The use of biofeedback has become increasingly important in the treatment of chronic pain. Biofeedback is a useful tool for reducing discomfort and enhancing overall well-being in patients by teaching them to identify and regulate physiological reactions connected to pain. The underlying tenet of biofeedback-based chronic pain management is that people can better regulate how they perceive and react to pain by increasing their awareness of their bodies' physiological cues.

Sensors are used in biofeedback techniques to track a variety of physiological data, including skin conductance, heart rate, muscle tension, and skin temperature. These measures can identify patterns of pain-related physiological reactions, some of which may be subconscious. Patients are given techniques to intentionally change these responses after these patterns are recognized. For instance, tension in the muscles and elevated stress levels can aggravate persistent musculoskeletal pain.

To ease pain and reduce muscle tension, patients can learn progressive muscle relaxation, deep breathing, and relaxation techniques with the aid of biofeedback.

Pain or discomfort coming from the muscles, bones, tendons, ligaments, and other connective tissues is referred to as musculoskeletal pain. Numerous illnesses, including fibromyalgia, arthritis, sprains of the muscles, and overuse injuries, can cause it. Since biofeedback can specifically target the physiological reactions that lead to pain, it is very helpful in the therapy of musculoskeletal pain.

By giving patients access to real-time data on muscular tension which frequently plays a major role in musculoskeletal pain biofeedback can assist patients with this kind of discomfort. Patients have control over their muscle activity and can monitor it with the help of electromyography (EMG) devices. After that, they can learn how to relax their muscles and ease discomfort by practicing biofeedback-assisted muscle relaxation, mental imagery, and relaxation techniques. By using these methods, people can become more adept at managing their pain and, in some situations, become less dependent on painkillers.

HEADACHES AND MIGRAINES

Migraines and tension headaches are prevalent, frequently incapacitating types of pain that are commonly accompanied by symptoms including light and sound sensitivity, nausea, and throbbing migraines. People with tension headaches and migraines have found that biofeedback is a useful supplementary therapy. It aids in the identification and management of the physiological variables that cause or worsen these headaches for patients.

In biofeedback sessions for managing migraines and headaches, sensors track variables such as muscle tension, skin temperature, and blood flow.

The goal of biofeedback practitioners is to assist patients in identifying precursors to and causes of their headaches. Through the recognition of patterns in their body's reactions, patients can learn to take action before a headache gets worse. Biofeedback methods to regulate blood vessel constriction and muscular tension—common factors leading to migraines and tension headaches include temperature biofeedback, relaxation training, and stress management approaches.

Biofeedback is a flexible therapeutic strategy that has important uses in the treatment of chronic pain, such as musculoskeletal pain and migraines. Biofeedback can dramatically enhance people's general well-being and lessen their need for painkillers by giving them more control over their physiological reactions. People looking for non-invasive, drug-free ways to properly treat chronic pain may find it to be a compelling choice.

RELAXATION TECHNIQUES

Stress and anxiety management is greatly aided by the use of relaxation techniques. These techniques cover a range of approaches meant to ease the body and quiet the mind. Among the often employed relaxation methods are progressive muscle relaxation, deep breathing exercises, awareness, and meditation. To reduce stress and promote relaxation, practice deep breathing by taking slow, deep breaths. The goal of progressive muscle relaxation is to release tension by gradually tensing and relaxing various muscle groups. By encouraging a greater awareness of the present moment, mindfulness and meditation help people break free from stressful thoughts and feelings. These methods offer a manner of self-regulation and emotional well-being, making them useful tools for people looking to reduce stress and anxiety.

STRESS-RELATED AILMENTS

Stress can cause several mental and physical stress-related ailments. Depression, panic disorder, post-traumatic stress disorder (PTSD), and generalized anxiety disorder are a few of these ailments. Physical illnesses brought on by stress might show up as gastrointestinal troubles, immune system dysfunction, and cardiovascular problems. Stress management is essential for general health and well-being since chronic stress can lead to the onset and aggravation of various conditions. It is frequently necessary to combine treatment modalities, such as psychotherapy, medication, and lifestyle changes to lower stress levels, to treat problems connected to stress.

ATTENTION AND FOCUS

An individual's capacity to sustain attention and focus can be greatly impacted by stress and worry. Stress causes the brain to redirect its cognitive resources toward the perceived threat, which makes it challenging to focus on information or tasks. Decision-making difficulties, memory problems, and lower productivity can all be consequences of this cognitive shift. Stress-reduction methods like mindfulness and meditation, as well as setting up a relaxing workplace with few distractions and stressors, are strategies to improve focus and attention. Additionally, leading a healthy lifestyle that includes regular exercise and a balanced diet can improve cognitive function and attentiveness.

ADHD AND BIOFEEDBACK

The neurodevelopment disorder known as Attention Deficit Hyperactivity Disorder (ADHD) is typified by issues with impulse control and attention maintenance. For those with ADHD, biofeedback is showing promise as a supplemental therapy. To offer real-time feedback, it entails monitoring physiological processes including heart rate, muscle tension, and brainwave patterns.

Controlling these physiological processes can help people with ADHD become more focused and self-reliant. People can improve their attention span and learn to adjust their brainwave activity with the use of biofeedback techniques like neurofeedback. Biofeedback is not an effective treatment for ADHD on its own, but it can be a useful part of a larger program.

PEAK PERFORMANCE

Depending on how they are handled, stress and anxiety can either prevent or help people function at their best. "Eustress," or a certain amount of stress, can improve performance and serve as motivation. On the other hand, excessive stress and worry, sometimes called "distress," can hinder optimal performance by raising bodily tension and affecting cognitive function. Understanding the ideal stress level for a given work or circumstance and using stress management strategies to stay within that range are necessary for achieving peak performance. By successfully controlling stress and anxiety, people can realize their full potential with the use of strategies like goal-setting, visualization, and encouraging self-talk.

Stress has a major role in the development of hypertension, or high blood pressure, which raises the risk of cardiovascular illnesses. Stress hormones that are released as a result of prolonged stress can narrow blood vessels, quicken the heartbeat, and ultimately raise blood pressure. This can deteriorate the arteries over time, raising the risk of heart attacks and strokes. Controlling stress is essential for heart health. A balanced diet, regular exercise, and stress-reduction methods like yoga and meditation can all help maintain healthy blood pressure levels and lower the risk of heart-related problems.

LOWERING BLOOD PRESSURE

Keeping blood pressure down is crucial for maintaining cardiovascular health overall. This can be done by combining medication and lifestyle changes. A heart-healthy diet reduced in sodium and saturated fats, frequent exercise, giving up smoking, and moderation in alcohol consumption are examples of lifestyle modifications. The use of stress-reduction strategies like mindfulness and relaxation training can also significantly lower blood pressure. Medication may be required in some cases to treat hypertension, however, for best effects, it is recommended to combine medication with lifestyle modifications.

HEART RATE VARIABILITY BIOFEEDBACK

The autonomic nervous system affects the heart rate variability biofeedback technique, which focuses on the fluctuation in time between subsequent heartbeats. It has drawn interest as a technique for reducing stress and enhancing general wellness. People can become more resilient to stress and enhance their cardiovascular health by increasing their heart rate variability. To achieve coherence between heart rate and breathing, this biofeedback approach entails modulating breathing patterns. With continued use, this technique can assist people in lowering their blood pressure, reducing stress, and improving their general well-being. An increasing number of people are using heart rate variability biofeedback in addition to conventional stress management and cardiovascular health techniques.

CHAPTER FIVE

THE METHOD OF BIOFEEDBACK

Through the use of real-time monitoring and feedback, the biofeedback process is a therapeutic strategy that enables people to take control of various physiological systems. The initial assessment, patient evaluation, goal-setting, training and practice, biofeedback techniques, biofeedback protocols, homework, and reinforcement are usually the main components of this procedure. We will go into great detail about each of these components to give you a clear idea of how biofeedback can be used as a useful therapeutic tool.

FIRST ASSESSMENT

Since it establishes the framework for the entire treatment plan, the first assessment is an essential stage in the biofeedback process. In this stage, the patient and the biofeedback practitioner collaborate closely to get pertinent data regarding the patient's medical background, present symptoms, and objectives. By using this information, the practitioner can better understand the unique requirements and concerns of the patient and adjust the biofeedback program as necessary.

PATIENT EVALUATION

A thorough patient evaluation is carried out after the initial assessment. Assessing the patient's physiological functions that are pertinent to the particular condition being treated is part of this examination. Depending on the patient's requirements, this may entail keeping an eye on variables including heart rate, breathing, skin conductance, muscle tension, and more. The assessment enables the healthcare provider to determine the patient's physiological reactions as a baseline and pinpoint areas in need of improvement.

ESTABLISHING SPECIFIC AND ACHIEVABLE GOALS FOR BIOFEEDBACK THERAPY

Following the completion of the initial assessment and patient evaluation, this is the following stage. The patient and the practitioner usually work together to define these objectives. The objectives can be very different and could involve controlling anxiety, reducing stress, managing pain, or enhancing general well-being. Establishing clear, quantifiable, and achievable objectives is crucial for monitoring advancement during the biofeedback procedure.

INSTRUCTION AND PRACTICE

Instruction and Practice include educating the patient on the proper way to operate biofeedback equipment and giving advice on how to accomplish the desired physiological changes. By watching real-time data on a computer screen or other feedback device, patients can learn to control their body systems. To modify physiological reactions, such as lowering heart rate, relaxing tense muscles, or raising skin temperature, the practitioner helps the patient develop the necessary skills and methods. To become proficient at these methods, you must practice them often.

BIOFEEDBACK TECHNIQUES

A range of approaches aimed at assisting patients in taking charge of their physiological processes are included in biofeedback techniques. These methods can involve gradual muscular relaxation, guided imagery, mindfulness meditation, and deep breathing exercises, among others. The patient's unique condition, goals, preferences, and degree of comfort with various methods all play a role in the strategies used.

Biofeedback protocols are customized treatment regimens that specify the methods, constraints, and objectives unique to each patient. These guidelines are created in consultation with the patient and are frequently modified in light of the patient's development. The frequency and length of biofeedback sessions may also be included in protocols, guaranteeing that the patient receives organized and constant assistance during the course of treatment.

ASSIGNMENTS AND REINFORCEMENT

To optimize the advantages of biofeedback, patients are usually given assignments and reinforcement exercises. This could entail using biofeedback techniques in everyday life or at home. Patients can continue to improve outside of the treatment setting by completing homework assignments that support the integration of newly acquired abilities into daily routines. Frequent follow-up meetings with the practitioner offer support, direction, and the chance to discuss any difficulties or roadblocks that may arise.

The biofeedback process is a methodical and cooperative strategy that empowers patients to actively participate in controlling their physiological reactions and enhancing their quality of life. To obtain positive outcomes, it entails several steps including the first assessment, patient evaluation, goal-setting, training, and practice, as well as the use of various biofeedback techniques, tailored biofeedback protocols, continuous homework, and reinforcement. Through self-regulation and self-awareness, individuals can increase their physical and mental health through this comprehensive approach that addresses a wide range of problems.

CHAPTER SIX

PROGRESS TRACKING AND MODIFICATIONS

Whether it is in the context of psychotherapy, healthcare, or any other type of intervention, progress monitoring and modifications are essential elements of any successful treatment plan. To keep the treatment plan in line with the patient's changing requirements and objectives, this process entails ongoing assessment, review, and change. Within this framework, several important ideas become essential components to take into account: monitoring outcomes, modifying the treatment plan, merging biofeedback with other therapies, integrative medicine, and psychiatric therapies.

MONITORING OUTCOMES

The core of progress monitoring is result tracking. This entails obtaining information and evaluating the results of a certain intervention. Measuring changes in vital signs, blood test results, or other physiological markers is one application of this in the healthcare industry. Monitoring psychotherapy progress might involve assessing behavioral or mood shifts as well as the accomplishment of certain treatment objectives. Healthcare professionals and therapists can determine if a treatment is beneficial, needs to be modified, or should be continued as is with the use of ongoing data collecting and analysis.

MODIFYING THE COURSE OF TREATMENT

One of the most important steps in the progress monitoring process is to modify the treatment plan. It recognizes that people are dynamic and that throughout time, their needs and reactions to treatments may vary. It is crucial to be adaptable and ready to change the treatment strategy as circumstances dictate. To better meet the patient's changing needs, this modification may entail modifying prescription drugs, therapy approaches, or lifestyle advice.

BLENDING BIOFEEDBACK WITH OTHER TREATMENT APPROACHES

Utilizing cutting-edge technologies and holistic health approaches is one strategy for combining biofeedback with other therapies. Through the use of biofeedback, people can become more conscious of and in control of their physiological functions, such as heart rate, blood pressure, and muscle tension. Patients can acquire the self-regulation abilities necessary to handle stress, pain, or a variety of medical disorders by incorporating biofeedback with conventional medical or psychological therapy. By treating the mental and physical facets of health, this integrative approach can increase the treatment plan's overall efficacy.

COMPLEMENTARY MEDICINE

Integrative medicine places a strong emphasis on providing healthcare as a whole. It addresses a person's mental, emotional, and social well-being in addition to their physical problems by fusing mainstream treatment with complementary and alternative therapies.

This method acknowledges that a person's health is impacted by several interrelated elements and that each should be taken into account in a thorough treatment plan. Integrative medicine promotes cooperation between many medical professionals to develop a comprehensive and unique treatment plan that enhances the patient's general health.

PSYCHOLOGIC INTERVENTIONS

In the context of mental health, psychological therapies are an essential part of progress monitoring and modifications. These treatments cover a broad spectrum of techniques, such as mindfulness-based therapies, psychoanalysis, and cognitive-behavioral therapy. They are crucial in assisting people in overcoming obstacles related to their mental health, enhancing their emotional health, and creating plans for self-improvement. By evaluating changes in behaviors, symptoms, and the attainment of therapeutic objectives, progress in psychological therapies is tracked, enabling therapists to modify their approaches to better suit the patient's needs.

The effectiveness of any treatment plan, whether it be in the medical or psychological realm, depends on progress monitoring and modifications.

A more thorough and patient-centered approach involves monitoring progress, making adjustments to the treatment plan, integrating biofeedback with other therapies, accepting integrated medicine, and using psychological therapies. Healthcare professionals and therapists may guarantee that the care they provide is customized to the evolving needs and objectives of the people they serve by regularly evaluating and modifying interventions. This will ultimately improve the health and well-being of the patients they serve.

CHAPTER SEVEN

BIOFEEDBACK IN PARTICULAR GROUPS

A useful treatment strategy that may be customized to fit the requirements of a variety of particular populations, such as kids and teenagers, senior citizens, athletes, and entertainers, is biofeedback. By giving people access to real-time data on physiological processes like heart rate, skin temperature, muscle tension, or brainwave activity, people can utilize this technology to become more conscious of and in control of their bodies. We will examine the uses of biofeedback in each of these distinct demographics in this talk.

CHILDREN & ADOLESCENTS AND BIOFEEDBACK

Biofeedback has the potential to be a useful therapeutic technique for children and adolescents, especially when it comes to stress, anxiety, and attention difficulties. Since young people frequently have trouble controlling their emotions and conduct, biofeedback is a useful technique for teaching self-regulation. They can learn how to control these reactions and acquire an understanding of how their bodies react to stimuli. Because it enhances focus and self-control, biofeedback might be especially beneficial for kids and teenagers with disorders like attention deficit hyperactivity disorder (ADHD).

APPLICATIONS IN PEDIATRICS

Biofeedback has the potential to alleviate several ailments in pediatric patients, such as chronic pain, anxiety problems, and asthma. Children who suffer from asthma, for example, can utilize biofeedback to enhance their breathing patterns and lessen the frequency and intensity of asthma episodes. Furthermore, the use of biofeedback techniques in therapy helps improve emotional regulation and self-awareness in children diagnosed with autism spectrum disorders.

CHILD-FRIENDLY WAYS

To pique children's and adolescents' attention and foster cooperation, it is imperative to employ child-friendly ways. To make the biofeedback process more engaging and intelligible for the younger participants, this may entail adding games, vibrant graphics, and interactive software into the sessions. Therapists can more effectively promote compliance and assist kids and teenagers in achieving great results by incorporating enjoyable and engaging elements into biofeedback sessions.

BIOFEEDBACK FOR SENIORS

When it comes to tackling age-related concerns like stress management and cognitive decline, biofeedback can be particularly helpful for senior citizens. Biofeedback is a useful tool for enhancing memory, cognitive function, and general mental health in older adults, as cognitive decline is a major problem.

GERIATRIC APPLICATIONS

By teaching relaxation techniques, encouraging better sleep, and lessening pain perception, biofeedback can assist older persons with a range of medical issues, such as arthritis, hypertension, and chronic pain. Through the provision of immediate feedback on physiological parameters, biofeedback enables senior citizens to actively participate in their healthcare and enhance their quality of life in general.

COGNITIVE DECLINE AND DEMENTIA

With the aging population growing, it is more crucial than ever to treat cognitive decline and dementia. Neurofeedback is one biofeedback approach that has demonstrated the potential to improve cognitive functioning in dementia patients. These methods try to help people with cognitive impairments with their memory, focus, and emotional control.

BIOFEEDBACK FOR PERFORMERS AND ATHLETES

Performers and athletes frequently have to meet high physical and psychological demands. Biofeedback can help them perform better and deal with problems like stage fright and nervousness when speaking in front of an audience.

IMPROVING SPORTS PERFORMANCE

By giving players more control over physiological functions like breathing, heart rate, and muscle tension, biofeedback is utilized to maximize sports performance. Athletes can learn how to maintain the ideal physiological condition for maximum performance and can monitor their stress levels.

This can enhance concentration, stamina, and the capacity to function under duress.

STAGE FRIGHT AND PUBLIC SPEAKING ANXIETY:

Performers and public speakers frequently struggle with stage fright and public speaking anxiety. By controlling heart rate, providing relaxation techniques, and lowering performance anxiety, biofeedback can benefit people working in various industries. Biofeedback gives performers control over their tension and anxiety so they may confidently provide their finest performances by giving them real-time data on physiological responses.

Biofeedback provides a flexible and adaptable strategy for a range of particular groups. Its uses include improving the performance of athletes and performers as well as assisting children and adolescents with self-regulation and cognitive decline in older persons.

CHAPTER EIGHT

MAKING USE OF BIOFEEDBACK

LOCATING A BIOFEEDBACK PRACTITIONER

To treat a variety of medical or psychological disorders, biofeedback therapy requires the assistance of a trained and experienced biofeedback therapist. In biofeedback therapy, physiological parameters including heart rate, skin temperature, and muscular tension are tracked and people are given real-time feedback on how their bodies are responding. By providing people with more control over these processes, this knowledge may enhance their overall health and well-being.

To include biofeedback treatment in one's medical regimen, finding a biofeedback therapist can be an important first step. Finding a therapist who has had biofeedback training and certification is crucial. To become certified biofeedback practitioners, a large number of healthcare professionals, such as psychologists, nurses, and physical therapists, must complete specific training. You might seek suggestions or references to licensed practitioners from your primary care physician or mental health provider to begin your search for a biofeedback therapist.

The Association for Applied Psychophysiology and Biofeedback (AAPB) and the Biofeedback Certification International Alliance (BCIA) are valuable resources for locating a biofeedback therapist. It is made simpler to find a licensed therapist in your region by using the directories of certified biofeedback practitioners maintained by these organizations. To find practitioners by area, area of expertise, or kind of certification, go to their websites.

SELECTING THE APPROPRIATE THERAPIST

It's critical to choose the best biofeedback therapist for your needs after you've found probable candidates. Take into account the following aspects to make an informed choice:

1. Qualifications and Certification: Check the therapist's credentials and make sure their certification is from an accredited body such as the BCIA. Their proficiency with biofeedback techniques is attested to by this accreditation.

2. Experience: Find out whether the therapist has dealt with any conditions comparable to yours before. It might be easier for a therapist with relevant experience to customize the biofeedback treatment to meet your needs.

3. Specialization: Certain biofeedback therapists focus on managing specific conditions, like pain, and tension, or improving athletic performance. Select a therapist whose skills complement your objectives.

4. Treatment Plan: Talk about the suggested course of action from the therapist. They ought to be able to outline the results you might anticipate

as well as how biofeedback will fit into your larger healthcare plan.

5. Compatibility: Establishing a solid therapeutic alliance is essential. Selecting a therapist with whom you are at ease and confident can improve the biofeedback therapy's efficacy.

6. Cost and Insurance: Find out how much biofeedback therapy will cost and if your insurance will pay for it. Be aware of any potential out-of-pocket costs so that you may choose wisely.

7. Location and Accessibility: Since you'll need to attend sessions regularly, take into account the therapist's location and accessibility. To make sure you can follow the suggested treatment plan, pick a convenient location.

PROSPECTIVE ADVANCEMENTS IN BIOFEEDBACK:

The field of biofeedback therapy is always changing in tandem with advancements in science and technology. Several fascinating upcoming advancements could improve the accessibility and efficacy of biofeedback therapy.

1. Wearable Biofeedback Devices: With the rise of wearable technology, like biosensors and smart watches, biofeedback may become more commonplace. These gadgets enable people to control stress, enhance well-being, and maximize performance by monitoring physiological data and providing real-time feedback.

2. Biofeedback in Virtual Reality (VR): Combining biofeedback with VR environments can produce therapeutic experiences that are fully immersive. This method exposes patients to regulated, therapeutic circumstances, which can be very helpful in treating disorders including anxiety, phobias, and post-traumatic stress disorder.

3. Personalized Biofeedback Apps: It's expected that there will be an increase in the use of mobile applications that are customized to a user's

requirements and preferences. With the use of guided biofeedback sessions, these apps can assist users in monitoring and enhancing physiological responses including skin conductance and heart rate variability.

4. Biofeedback in Telehealth: Biofeedback therapy may become more widely available as telehealth services grow. People who would like to undergo biofeedback therapy from the comforts of their homes can do so with the help of remote monitoring and video conversations.

5. The use of biofeedback to supplement conventional mental health therapies is gaining traction in the field of mental health. As research in this area progresses, biofeedback might become increasingly important in treating ailments like attention deficit disorder, anxiety, and depression.

6. Integration of Biofeedback in Sports and Performance: To maximize their physical and

mental potential, athletes and people aiming for top performance are increasingly utilizing biofeedback. Future advancements might include training methods to improve sports performance and recuperation as well as more advanced biofeedback instruments.

The first step in utilizing this beneficial type of therapy is to locate a biofeedback therapist. Making sure the therapist is qualified and choosing the best expert for your needs are important factors to take into account. Furthermore, biofeedback has a bright future ahead of it thanks to technological breakthroughs and creative applications that will broaden its use and increase its efficacy across a range of healthcare and well-being domains.